INTERMITTENT

FASTING OVER 50

for Women

30-Days Meal Plan

100 RECIPES

The Ultimate Guide of Anti-Aging Solutions Recharge Energy and Memory, Improve Your Health and Correct Metabolism
Lose Weight

2024

I0792052

\+ health tracker

Juliya Jones

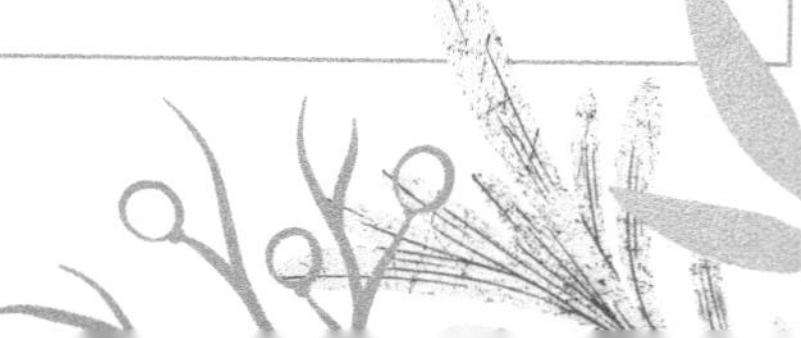

Table of Contents

Table of Contents

Table of Contents

Introduction

A brief introduction to intermittent fasting and its health benefits

Have you ever heard of interval fasting (IF)? It's not just another trendy thing in the health and fitness world; it's a real game changer in the approach to nutrition and weight management. People love it, and here's why.

Imagine this: You can eat and lose weight. It's like a dream, wouldn't you say? Intermittent fasting not only makes this possible, but it will also help you look 5–10 years younger.

It's not about torturing yourself with hunger strikes; it's about choosing a time to eat that works best for your body and lifestyle. And yes, you can enjoy your favorite foods at these times and still feel a surge of energy and strength at the same time.

Fears: forget them!

Many people are frightened when they hear the word "fasting." "Do I really have to abstain from food and torture myself?" they ask. The answer is no!

It's not about starving yourself; it's about eating your daily ration for a short period of time. It's not about restricting food; it's about adjusting the timing of your food intake.

The benefits are many!

During intermittent fasting, you lose weight, get rid of old, damaged cells, and replace them with young, new cells, but you also get other visible health benefits.

Insulin sensitivity is improved, and this is important for diabetes prevention. Inflammation levels tend to drop, making IF strong in the fight against diseases like obesity, cancer, and Alzheimer's. It's also a great way to strengthen the heart and brain, rejuvenate blood vessels, and normalize blood pressure, prolonging youthfulness and activity.

Schedule it when you need it!

One of the great things about IF is its flexibility. You can choose the fasting schedule that best fits your lifestyle. Whether it's 16/8, where you eat for 8 hours and fast for 16, or 5/2, where you restrict calories "two days,"

It's your choice, and you can change it based on your goals.

Plus, many people find that that interval fasting is just convenient. Forget lugging around three containers of food or worrying about finding a healthy lunch at the office. You just eat when it's convenient for you and give your body a break the rest of the time.

So if you're thinking about interval fasting, if you can see the potential for yourself, why not give it a try? Who knows, it could be just what your body and brain need!

Overview of the main components of the book

Introduction to Interval Fasting (16:8)

We start with the basics. This is like our warm-up before the main marathon. Here you'll learn what interval fasting is, what the most popular regimen is, and how to properly divide your day into periods of eating and fasting. This will help you prepare for changes in your diet and life without feeling lost in the Three Pines.

Meal Frequency

This is about how often you're going to eat in those same 8 hours. This is important so you don't feel hungry and your metabolism works like a Swiss watch. You'll also learn how to spread those meals out so you have enough energy to last all day.

Managing Insulin for Weight Loss

As you age, your body's insulin levels can work against you. Here we show you how to improve them and even lose weight with intermittent fasting and proper nutrition. It's like finding a second youth without resorting to magic.

Nutrient Absorption

Not all calories are equal, right? We'll teach you how to choose foods that not only taste good but also do the most good for your body. It's like choosing between a fast carbohydrate and a complex carbohydrate that will give you an instant boost, while the other will keep you feeling energized for a long time.

Meal Plans and Recipes

This is the heart of the book! There are over 100 recipes to help you not only lose weight but also enjoy every meal.

It's like having a personal chef, except you're behind the stove.

Vitamins and Foods for Weight Loss

Here we dive into the world of vitamins and minerals your body needs for health and longevity. It's like a cocktail of the healthiest ingredients to help your body function at peak performance and burn extra calories like a real fitness trainer.

Chapter 1: Introduction to Interval Fasting

The Science Behind IF: How It Works and How It Affects Your Body

Do you want to learn about interval fasting (IF) and its effects on your body? I will explain it to you simply, without any complications.

Think of your body as a perfect machine that can run on different types of fuel. Normally, we give it glucose from the food we eat.

During intermittent fasting, the body turns to its fat reserves for energy.

During intermittent fasting, the body turns to its fat reserves for energy. This process is comparable to discovering a piggy bank full of money when your wallet is empty. It feels satisfying.

In addition, fasting can lower blood insulin levels, which promotes the burning of fat for energy and can result in weight loss without any external intervention.

Additionally, when you refrain from eating, your body undergoes a process known as autophagy. During this process, your cells eliminate old and damaged components, which can help prevent various diseases such as cancer and memory loss. Autophagy can be likened to thorough housecleaning for your body.

Another benefit of practicing IF is the increase in growth hormone levels in your body. This hormone aids in muscle building and fat burning, while also slowing down the aging process. Therefore, it can be said that IF promotes weight loss and contributes to a more youthful appearance.

Overall, intermittent fasting is not solely focused on weight loss, but also on improving health, energy, and potentially longevity. The best part is that it is simple to begin - decide when to eat and when to rest your body. There are no strict diets, calorie counting, or torture involved. Simply live and enjoy the process.

Different types of IF plans (16/8, 5/2, OMAD) and how to choose the right one for you

"All right, guys, let's go."

All right guys, let's get all these interval fasting modes sorted out, because there is a choice, and it's not a small one!

16/8

This is the classic of the genre. 16 hours of no-never, then eat whatever you want for 8 hours, it's like the new hit among diets. Well, within reason of course. Suitable for those who want to make IF their lifestyle without much upheaval. You skip breakfast and enjoy lunch and dinner. Perfect for beginners.

For example, eat breakfast at noon and lock up the kitchen at 8 pm. And that's every day.

That means your dinner and breakfast the next day are separated by a full 16 hours of pure fasting.

What's cool about that? Well, for one thing, it gives your body time to take a break from constantly processing food. During this time, processes like fat burning and detoxification can kick in because the body isn't busy digesting fresh calories.

Also, many people find that it becomes easier to control the total number of calories consumed on this diet - simply because there is less time to eat.

The second benefit is flexibility. You choose when your 8-hour eating
window begins. Many people like to skip breakfast and start eating at lunch, but others prefer to eat a solid breakfast and end the day with an early dinner.

But remember, it's not just when you eat, it's what you eat. The 16/8 diet doesn't give you carte blanche to eat anything you want. To make it work for your health and figure, you need to choose nutritious foods that give you energy and don't leave you feeling hungry an hour after you eat.

So if you're looking for a way to tweak your diet and give your body more time to recover, the 16/8 diet could be your option. Just remember to watch the quality of your food and don't turn your "meal windows" into unbridled feasts every day!

5/2

The 5/2 diet is kind of your trick in the weight loss world, suggested by Dr. Michael Mosley from the UK. He picked up on the idea - not total starvation, but you just cut down to 500-600 calories a day for two days a week, and live the other five days as normal.

That way you trigger a bunch of cool bodily processes similar to what happens when you don't eat at all. This diet is for those who aren't ready to starve themselves every day but are willing to kick their habits a few times a week.

You can spread these two days out however you like - at least back to back, at least spread out throughout the week. The idea is to make it less excruciating because going completely without food for an entire day is an unrealistically difficult task for many people.

So here's a doctor's tip for you: cut back on calories, but don't starve yourself completely. And it's not a one-time thing. Once you've reached your desired weight, stick with it so you don't lose the results.

People like Stella from Leeds say it's okay to skip a few meals and that most of the fasting is done at bedtime, so it's not that hard. Oh, and food seems to taste better on fasting days because you're hungry.

Mark Sisson, another fan of fasting, says that for those who want to lose a lot of extra weight and are already used to burning fat, try fasting for 24, 36, or even 48 hours at a time. The key is to remember to be physically active so that the body burns fat and uses ketones

OMAD (One Meal A Day)

For the most resilient. It's simple: one meal a day and that's it. This option gives you the maximum fasting time, but man, does it require an iron will?

If you can get through the daydreaming of that one, but very nutritious and delicious meal, why not?

How to choose?

You should choose based on your lifestyle, preferences, and goals. If you're a beginner, start with 16/8 - it's the mildest option. If you like to experiment and are ready for more, try 5/2 or even OMAD.

The most important rule is to listen to your body. If you feel something is not right, you can try a different regimen or adjust your current one. There is no one right way for everyone, to each his own.

And remember folks, intermittent fasting is not a short-term diet, it is a lifestyle. It's not about hunger, it's about freedom from constant snacking and the ability to feel real hunger and enjoy food. And yes, the benefits can be achieved without cost, without drugs or vitamin supplements. Just choose your path and choose health and longevity!

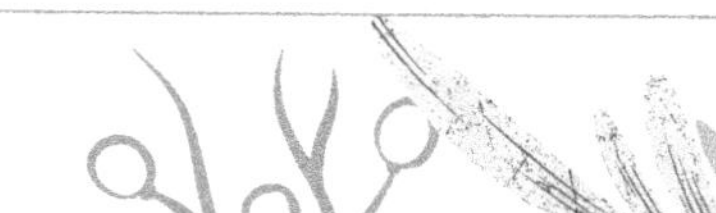

Aligning with the Body's Circadian Rhythms

Let's talk about circadian rhythms and how they relate to interval fasting. It sounds like science fiction, but it's quite simple.

Circadian rhythms are your body's internal clock. They regulate a whole host of things, from when you want to sleep to how your metabolism processes food. And it turns out that when you eat in sync with these rhythms, your body runs like a Swiss watch.

By default, our bodies prefer to be active and eat during the day when it's light, and rest at night when it's dark. So when you do interval fasting and choose to eat during daylight hours, like 10 am to 6 pm, it's like you're telling your internal clock, "Hey, it's okay, we're working on schedule.

This alignment with circadian rhythms not only helps you better burn calories and manage your appetite, but it also promotes better sleep. And a good night's sleep is half the success of any diet or health improvement plan, right? When you get a good night's sleep, your brain and body repair, regenerate, and prepare for the new day.

So when you eat according to your circadian rhythms, you help your body make the most efficient use of food, reduce your risk of weight gain, and improve your overall health.

It's like synchronizing your internal clock with nature's cycle of light and darkness and betting on your health and well-being.

In general, when choosing a time frame for interval fasting, think about your natural rhythms. If you're an owl, it might make sense to move your eating window a little later, and if you're a lark, start and end earlier. The key is to make sure it works with your lifestyle and circadian rhythms. This will help you get the most out of interval fasting and take another step towards health and longevity!

The Role of Autophagy in Aging and Disease Prevention

Okay, let's talk more about something super cool, the process of autophagy.
Autophagy, folks, is our internal cleaning service that runs 24/7 but is turned on full blast during interval fasting. Imagine little workers inside your body cleaning up all the junk, old, and damaged particles, and making room for new ones. It's not magic, it's science!

Autophagy and Aging

As we age, our internal cleaning service starts to slow down. Autophagy helps "rejuvenate" cells by ridding them of "aging junk". Less junk means slower aging. It's like regularly updating your smartphone to keep it running like new. So autophagy is a refresh for your cells.

Autophagy and disease prevention

When the body gets rid of cellular waste, it reduces the risk of many diseases. Cancer, Alzheimer's, cardiovascular disease - all of these problems can be linked to the accumulation of damaged cells and proteins. Autophagy, on the other hand, helps "take out the trash" by preventing the accumulation of harmful materials.

Autophagy is like a repair

Imagine that your body is a house that needs to be repaired from time to time to keep everything nice and functional. Autophagy is like repairs that help keep the "house" in order and prevent its premature destruction; it is a process of cleaning the body at the cellular level.
So when you practice interval fasting and trigger autophagy, you are investing in your health and longevity. It doesn't require money, expensive drugs, or supplements. Just give your body a little break from food and it will thank you by cleaning up inside and protecting you from aging and disease.

All in all, fasting isn't just about weight loss, it's about self-care on a cellular level. So let's give this amazing process a try, and who knows, maybe we can cheat time and live happily ever after!

Chapter 2: A Strategy for Introducing Interval Fasting

A step-by-step guide to gradually incorporating fasting into your lifestyle

Let's look at how to start your interval fasting adventure without turning your life into a hellish ordeal. Everything should be done gently and smoothly so that you don't even notice how you've fallen in love with this lifestyle. Let's go step by step!

Step 1: Reconnaissance

Before you get started, spend a week simply observing your usual meal and snack times. Write down what you eat, when you eat it, and how you feel about it. This will give you an idea of what you're up against.

Step 2: Start small

Choose a shorter fasting window, such as 12 hours. This may sound like a lot, but if you're eating at 7 p.m. and having breakfast at 7 a.m., congratulations, you're on the right track! Gradually increase your fast to 14 hours, then 16 hours.

Step 3: Water is your best friend

Drink plenty of water during your fast. This will help you manage your hunger and improve your overall health. Herbal tea or black coffee is also fine, as long as it's without sugar or milk.

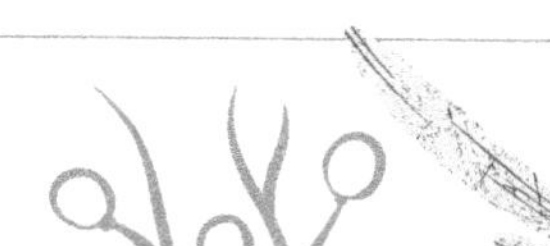

Step 4: Listen to your body

This is important. If you feel like you're not feeling well, it might be a good idea to eat a little. Interval fasting is not a competition. The goal is to improve your health, not to martyr yourself.

Step 5: Eat a balanced diet

When you do eat, try to focus on nutritious, balanced meals. Proteins, fats, carbohydrates, vitamins, and minerals should all be included in your diet. This will keep you full and energized.

Interval fasting is more of a marathon than a sprint. You shouldn't feel hungry or miserable all the time. On the contrary, it should give you pleasure and a sense of ease. So start slow, enjoy the process, and watch your body and mind thank you.

Tips to minimize discomfort and improve compliance

And here are a few lifehacks to make your journey into the world of interval fasting feel like you're on wings, without too many thorns in the way and with maximum enjoyment.

1. Start with taste

The first rule of the intermittent fasting club: don't make food the enemy. Choose tasty but healthy foods so that every meal is a small feast. That way, you'll look forward to and enjoy your meal window.

2. Smarts to watch for

If you're hungry during your fast, use your wits. Water, green tea, or black coffee without anything in it can be your best friends.

They will help "trick" your stomach and make you feel full. And yes, get some exercise: a walk or a short meditation works wonders.

3. Engage in your favorite activities

Find an activity that distracts you from thoughts of food. A book, a movie, a hobby - anything. If you're busy, your brain won't be spinning the same record about food.

4. Appropriate flexibility

Remember that strict discipline is good, but life is unpredictable. If you have to deviate from your schedule on any given day, don't beat yourself up. Just pick yourself up the next time with renewed vigor. It's the overall direction that matters, not the day-to-day victories.

5. Support is Key to Success

Find like-minded people or friends who are also doing interval fasting. Sharing experiences, support, and eating together during your meal window will make the process more enjoyable and easier.

6. Track your progress

Keeping a food and wellness journal is a great idea. This will help you track your progress, understand what works best, and adjust the plan to suit you.

Remember that the goal of intermittent fasting is not only weight loss, but also improved health, energy, and overall quality of life. So do your best to make the process enjoyable, not a burden. Be smart about it, listen to your body, and be prepared for each day to bring something new.

Chapter 3: Meal Frequency

Recommendations for the number of meals you should eat during an 8-hour window

Now it's time to talk about the most popular meal pattern for beginners, the 16/8 pattern, and how often you should eat during those eight hours when you can eat. This is important because proper meal distribution can make your interval fasting even more effective. So hang in there, we're going to break it all down.

Let's go point by point:

1. Start with balance

First and most importantly, don't try to eat your entire daily diet in one meal. You don't want to feel like a balloon, right? Aim for 2-3 meals within those 8 hours. This will help you stay full and give your body enough energy for the day.

2. Breakfast? Lunch? Dinner?

Let's say your eating window is from noon to 8 pm. It's ideal to start with lunch at noon, then have a light snack or second meal around 3 to 4 p.m., and finish with dinner at 7:30 p.m. This distribution gives you enough time to digest your food before your next meal and before your fast begins.

3. Snacking - yes or no?

If you feel hungry between main meals, light snacks are okay. But choose something healthy like nuts, yogurt, or fresh fruit. They'll help you stay energized and keep you from reaching for something less healthy.

4. Listen to your body

This is the golden rule for any eating plan, but it's especially important here. If you're not hungry, don't force yourself to eat just because it's "mealtime. Your body is your best advisor.

5. Planning is the key to success

Try to plan your meals and snacks ahead of time. This will help you avoid impulsive eating decisions and keep you on track.

6. Enjoy every bite

When you're eating, focus on the food. Enjoy the flavor, texture, and aroma of the food. Not only will this improve your mood, but it will also help you feel more satisfied.

And there you are a master of interval fasting, armed with the knowledge of how to spread out your meals.

Tips for Boosting Your Metabolism and Lowering Your Insulin Levels

Now that we've covered the frequency of eating, let's talk about how to make this ritual not only enjoyable but also as beneficial to your metabolism and insulin levels as possible. There are a few tricks that can help you keep things in check.

Here's how to make friends with your metabolism and insulin:

1. Protein and fiber to protect your metabolism

Include protein and fiber at every meal. Protein is the building block of your body, while fiber helps keep you feeling full longer and normalizes blood sugar levels. Avocados, nuts, whole grains, meat, fish, and legumes are your best friends.

2. "Smart" carbohydrates

Choose carbohydrates with a low glycemic index (GI), which raise blood sugar levels more slowly. You'll avoid insulin spikes. Sweet potatoes, quinoa, brown rice - these are the champions of energy stabilization.

3. Don't forget healthy fats

Olive oil, nuts, flaxseed, and of course omega-3 omega-3-rich fish. These foods not only support your brain and heart but also help regulate insulin levels and boost your energy.

4. Miracle Beverages

Green tea and coffee (no sugar or cream, of course) are your trusty companions in the fight for a dream metabolism. Not only do they help speed up your metabolism, but they can also lower your blood sugar levels slightly.

5. Mix up the calories

Play around with the number of calories you consume each day, don't let your body get used to the same daily amount. This can help speed up your metabolism because your body is constantly guessing how much to process.

6. Don't sit still

Even light physical activity throughout the day can help speed up your metabolism and control your insulin levels. You don't have to wait until after your meal, a short walk after your meal is a great idea.

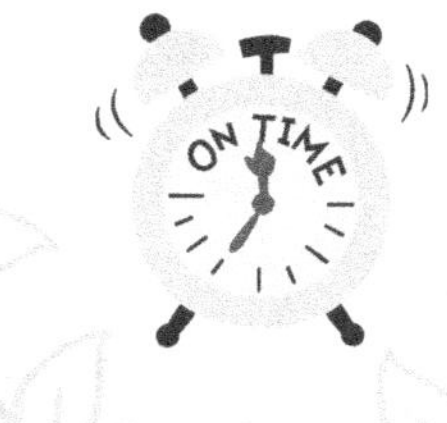

How Water Consumption Affects Metabolism and Weight Loss

Come on, speed up your metabolism and lose weight with...
water! Water! Yes, yes, don't be surprised, ordinary water can
be your true ally on the road to slimness. Here's how it works:

Water is a metabolism turbocharger

1. Boosts Metabolism: Imagine each sip of water is like a little
kick to your metabolism, telling it, "Come on, work faster!"
Studies have shown that drinking cold water can temporarily
increase your metabolic rate because it requires more energy to
bring it to body temperature.

2. Reduces appetite: Try drinking a glass of water 20-30
minutes before you eat. You may be surprised, but you'll feel
less hungry and eat less. Water helps "trick" your stomach into
feeling full without the extra calories.

Water is a liquid trainer

In addition to directly affecting your metabolism, water helps to
- Increase physical activity: Dehydration can hinder the effects
of exercise by causing weariness and a decrease in energy.
 Adequate water intake helps maintain optimal energy levels
and improves athletic performance.
- Get rid of toxins: Water helps the kidneys filter and eliminate

toxins from the body. Fewer toxins mean better metabolic function and easier weight loss.

How much to drink

Aiming for the recommended 8 glasses (roughly 2 liters) throughout the day is a good place to start, though there isn't a universally applicable recommendation.

"Drink when you feel thirsty" is the golden rule. But if you're active or it's hot outside, increase your water intake. Pay attention to your body's cues, such as the color of your urine—a pale yellow hue is a good sign of hydration.
And remember, fruits and vegetables can also help you stay hydrated.

The bottom line

So if you want to keep your metabolism going and speed up your weight loss, don't forget about water. It is the easiest, most accessible, and most importantly, free way to help yourself get healthier and slimmer. Drink water and be happy!

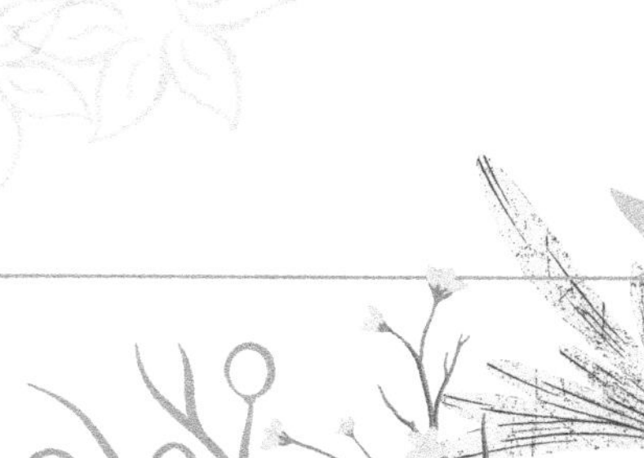

The Impact of Hydration on Energy Levels and Cognitive Function

So, folks, how many of you forget to drink water throughout the day? Admit it! You should, because hydration isn't just about skin health and weight loss. It's also about your energy and mental performance. Let's explain why water is so important to our brains and bodies.

Water for Energy: How Does It Work?

1. Happiness: Feeling low on energy? Before you run out for coffee, try drinking a glass of water. Even mild dehydration can make you feel tired and lethargic. Water helps your blood carry oxygen and nutrients to your cells, giving you more energy.

2. Endurance: For those who exercise, hydration is critical. Without enough water, your workouts will be harder and recovery will take longer. Drink up, folks, and you'll be glad you did!

Water and the Brain: Friends Forever

1. Concentration: Without enough water, your brain slows down. Having a water bottle on hand will help you stay productive and focused.

2. Memory and mood: Studies show dehydration negatively affects your memory and can cause irritability. Want to be in a good mood and remember where you left your keys? Drink water!

The bottom line

Staying hydrated is an easy way to keep yourself physically and mentally healthy. Don't wait until you feel thirsty, but sip water regularly throughout the day. Your body and brain will thank you for it. So let's make our next toast to health ..... with a glass of water!

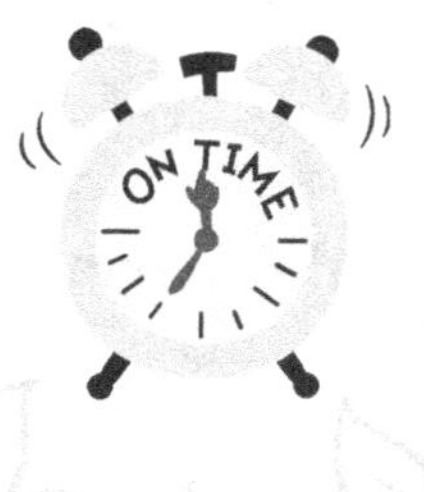

Chapter 4: Using Insulin for Weight Loss

The effects of insulin on weight and ways to reduce insulin resistance

Okay, let's break it down. All this hype about diets and weight loss, and it turns out it's not about calories. It's not about how much you eat or how much you waste, it's about what's going on in your body on a hormonal level.

Insulin is the hormone responsible for fat storage. When we eat, our insulin levels spike, telling our body, "We're storing fat for a rainy day. And if that rainy day never comes (because we keep eating and eating and eating), insulin continues to store fat that way.

All these years we've been told to eat less and exercise more. But it turns out that's not the answer. We've tried everything, and guess what? It doesn't work. The real problem with obesity is not eating too many calories, it is a hormonal malfunction.

Here's what you need to know to make insulin your ally:

1. Insulin and weight-what's the connection?

helps your body's cells absorb glucose from the blood for energy.

When there is too much sugar in the blood, the body produces more insulin to deal with it, and this can lead to fat storage, especially if the energy is not used. Therefore, the key to weight loss is to keep insulin levels normal to avoid storing extra fat.

2. Reduce Insulin Resistance

Insulin resistance is when your body's cells become less sensitive to insulin, and the body has to produce more of it to deal with glucose. This not only increases your risk of developing type 2 diabetes but also makes it harder to control your weight. A healthy diet, regular exercise, and weight control can help reduce insulin resistance.

3. Stabilizing Blood Sugar

Avoid blood sugar spikes by choosing foods with a low glycemic index. More fiber (vegetables, whole grains), less sugar, and refined carbohydrates. And yes, healthy fats and proteins should be your faithful companions at every meal.

4. Exercise is life

Exercise not only helps you burn calories, it also improves insulin sensitivity. Find something you enjoy: walking, running, swimming, yoga, or dancing. The key is to do it regularly.

5. Get sleep and stress under control

Lack of sleep and chronic stress can raise insulin and blood sugar levels, contributing to fat storage.

So quality sleep and stress management are your best friends in the fight for a slimmer figure.

Insulin and weight: what you need to know

When you eat, especially carbohydrates, blood sugar levels rise and the pancreas produces insulin to help cells absorb sugar (glucose) from the bloodstream. If there is too much sugar and it is constantly elevated, the body begins to produce more and more insulin to handle the load. Over time, this can lead to insulin resistance, where your body's cells become less sensitive to insulin. This, in turn, causes your body to store fat instead of using it for energy.

How to reduce insulin resistance

1. Cut back on carbohydrates

Start by reducing your intake of simple carbohydrates such as white bread, sweets, and soda. This will help lower your blood sugar levels and reduce your body's need for insulin.

2. Fiber is your friend

Fiber helps slow the absorption of sugar, which helps control blood sugar and insulin levels. Eat more vegetables, fruits, and whole grains!

3. Exercise regularly

Physical activity improves insulin sensitivity because muscles use glucose for energy during exercise, lowering blood glucose levels. Combine aerobic exercise with strength training for the best results.

4. Maintain a healthy weight

Losing excess weight, even if it's only 5-10% of your total body weight, can significantly improve insulin sensitivity and reduce your risk of developing type 2 diabetes.

5. Get enough sleep

Lack of sleep can lead to higher insulin and blood glucose levels, so don't forget to get a solid 7-8 hours of sleep.

6. Reduce stress

Stress causes the body to produce cortisol, which can raise sugar

Eating food 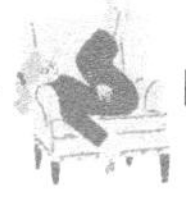 Insulin's going up 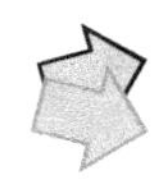 The liver stores sugar
The liver produces fat

Not eating food 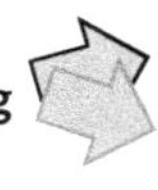 Insulin is dropping Sugar reserves burn off
Fat reserves are burned

Chapter 5: Nutrient Absorption

The Importance of Gut Health for Nutrient Absorption

So let's talk about something important, and that's gut health. This topic, friends, is cooler than any TV show because it's all about us and our well-being.

Think of the gut not as something unpleasant, but as your chef who cooks and serves you all the nutrients you need. When the chef is happy and healthy, the food is digested perfectly. But if he's upset, well, you know.

Why do we need a healthy gut?

1. Better absorption of nutrients: A healthy gut is key to making sure that all the vitamins, minerals, and antioxidants from your food get to where they need to go instead of just passing through. It's like having a super-efficient vacuum cleaner that doesn't leave a crumb behind.

2- Shield against the bad guys: Our gut is a barrier to harmful bacteria and toxins. When it's in good shape, bad guys don't stand a chance. It's like a wall protecting your castle from marauders.

3. Happy gut = happy brain: Did you know that most serotonin (the happy hormone) is made in the gut? So the health of your gut is directly linked to your mood. When the gut is happy, you're happy.

How do you keep your gut in tip-top shape?

- Food variety: The more diverse the beneficial bacteria in your gut, the stronger your digestive system. Feed them a variety of foods-vegetables, fruits, fermented milk.

- Prebiotics and probiotics: These are like food and friends for your gut bacteria. Prebiotics are found in whole grains, fruits, and vegetables, and probiotics are found in yogurt and other fermented foods.

- Reduce stress: Yes, stress affects gut health. So let's relax more and enjoy life.
So treat your gut like your best friend. If it is happy, you will be happy, healthy, and full of energy. It's like having a superhero on your team, ready to save the day. Go, gut!

Foods and Methods that Enhance Your Cells' Absorption of Nutrients

Okay, let's break down what gizmos and tricks help our cells absorb nutrients like a sponge absorbs water. After all, it's no secret that how and what we eat determines how much goodness our cells get.

Superhero Foods

1. Fatty fish: Contains omega-3 fatty acids, which not only make you smarter but also help you absorb vitamins A, D, E, and K. So salmon, mackerel, and sardines are your best friends.

2- Colorful fruits and vegetables: The carotenoids that make fruits and vegetables so colorful improve the absorption of antioxidants. Carrots, squash, and ripe tomatoes are all good for you.

3. Dairy products: The probiotics in yogurt or kefir not only keep your gut healthy but also help with nutrient absorption. Happy gut - happy cells.

Cooking methods and other tricks

1. Fermented foods: Kimchi, sauerkraut, and other fermented foods improve nutrient absorption and promote gut health.

2. Sprouting and soaking: Soaking beans, seeds, and grains helps eliminate phytic acid, which can interfere with mineral absorption. Sprouting increases the amount and availability of nutrients.

3. less processing, more benefits: The less processed a food is, the more nutrients it retains. So fans of chips and breadcrumbs should think twice.

4. The right combination of foods: Vitamin C improves the absorption of iron from plant foods. That's why a spinach salad with lemon juice is not only tasty but also healthy.

You also need to know that iron is poorly absorbed with calcium.
Iron and calcium are two important minerals for our bodies, but when they come together, there can be problems with assimilation.

The thing is that calcium can interfere with the absorption of iron. When consumed at the same time, calcium competes with iron for the "attention" of special molecules in the intestines that are responsible for absorption. As a result, the body absorbs less iron than it could.

This is especially important for people with iron deficiencies or those on vegetarian or vegan diets, where iron is mostly in a non-essential form that is already less absorbable than iron from meat products.

To minimize this conflict:

- Avoid eating dairy products with iron-rich foods. For example, if you have spinach salad (a source of iron) for lunch, don't wash it down with a glass of milk.

- You should also avoid taking calcium supplements with iron-rich foods or iron supplements. If you're taking both types of supplements, try to take them at different times of the day.

- Include vitamin C-rich foods in your diet along with iron sources - vitamin C helps improve iron absorption. For example, a fruit salad with strawberries or citrus fruits would be a good addition to a lentil dish.

- Avoid combining calcium-rich foods, such as cheese or yogurt, with iron-rich foods in the same meal.

Remember, balancing the absorption of these minerals is more a matter of careful planning than eliminating certain foods from your diet altogether.

In general, if you want your body to run like a Swiss watch, make friends with foods that enhance nutrient absorption, and don't forget the little tricks of preparation. Remember, our bodies are complex but amazing systems that will thank you for your care and attention. Eat right and enjoy life!

The Role of Intermittent Fasting in Improving Gut Health and Nutrient Absorption

So friends, let's talk about how intermittent fasting keeps our gut happy and helps our cells soak up all the good stuff from food like a sponge.

The Gut is Our Inner Garden

Think of the gut as a garden where beneficial bacteria grow. For the garden to be healthy, it needs a break from constantly digesting food. This is where intermittent fasting comes in. It gives our "garden" a break to recover and prepare for a new growing season.

Scavenging

When you don't eat for a few hours, your gut begins a general cleaning process to remove damaged cells and waste. This is called autophagy, which we've already talked about. A clean gut not only means good digestion but also better nutrient absorption.

How does this work?

When you give your body a break from eating, your insulin levels drop, which signals your gut to work on itself. Less inflammation, better microflora balance, and voila-nutrients are absorbed like clockwork.

Bonus: Hello, Good Bacteria

Starvation helps increase the amount of beneficial bacteria in your gut. These guys not only help us digest food, but they're also involved in vitamin production, infection defense, and even mood regulation. In essence, intermittent fasting is like handing out superfoods to our microbial friends.

The Bottom Line

Intermittent fasting isn't just a way to lose weight or improve your figure. It's really about gut health and better nutrient absorption. It's like giving your inner world a little rest so it can work even better for you.
So if you're looking for a way to improve your health from the inside out, don't forget about the magic of intermittent fasting. Your gut will thank you, and you'll feel the difference not only in your stomach but in your overall health. On to a healthy "garden"!

The Importance of Nutritious Foods and Preparing the Right Meals

Let's take a closer look at how to make each meal as beneficial to your body as possible so that nutrient absorption is at its highest. It's like creating the perfect food team, where everyone plays their part and helps each other perform better.

The secrets of a nutritious feast are

1- Balance is everything

Every meal you eat should be like a piece of art: a combination of proteins, fats, carbohydrates, and fiber. Protein supports your muscles, healthy fats improve vitamin absorption, carbohydrates give you energy, and fiber helps you digest. That's a four you can't do without.

2. Variety is the key to vitamins

You don't have to eat the same thing every day. A variety of foods ensures that you get all the micronutrients and vitamins you need. Think of your plate as an artist's palette: the more colorful and varied, the better.

3. "Whole foods come first

Focus on whole, unprocessed foods. They contain the most nutrients. Vegetables, fruits, whole grains, nuts, and seeds are your mainstays.

Processed foods often lose a lot of goodness in the manufacturing process and are loaded with unnecessary sugars and preservatives.

4. Proper heat processing

Some cooking methods can improve nutrient absorption, while others can make it worse. For example, lightly steaming vegetables makes some antioxidants more available for absorption. However overcooking or prolonged cooking can destroy beneficial substances.

5. Combining foods

Some foods, when eaten together, can enhance each other's benefits. For example, iron from plant sources is better absorbed when combined with vitamin C, so add some citrus or tomatoes to dishes with green leafy vegetables.

6. Pay Attention to Your Microbiota

The health of your gut has a direct impact on nutrient absorption. Foods rich in probiotics and fiber promote the growth of beneficial microflora and improve digestion and absorption. Foods like yogurt, kefir, sauerkraut, and fiber-rich fruits and vegetables are your allies in maintaining gut health. Eating these foods regularly can help you not only absorb nutrients better but also boost your immune system.

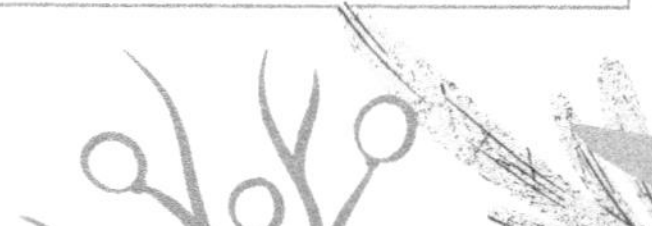

Here are a few more tips to get you started:

Listen to yourself

Your body is your best advisor. If you experience discomfort, bloating, or other unpleasant symptoms after eating certain foods, it may be time to rethink your diet. Not all seemingly healthy foods are right for everyone.

Variety is the key

Don't get stuck on the same foods. Variety not only keeps you from getting bored but also provides a wide range of nutrients. Experiment with different types of vegetables, fruits, proteins, fats, and carbohydrates.

Chew thoroughly

Remember that the digestion process starts in the mouth. Chewing thoroughly not only makes it easier on your stomach and intestines but also helps you absorb nutrients better. It also helps you enjoy the taste of your food and feel fuller.

Meal Planning

Try to plan your meals so that they are balanced and nutritious. Planning will help you avoid impulsive decisions in favor of quick, but not the healthiest, meals.
By investing a little time and attention in your diet, you can maximize the benefits of each meal and improve your health and well-being. It's like making an investment in yourself that's sure to pay off!

Chapter 6: 30–Day Meal Plan

30-Day Meal Plan

Okay, now that we've discussed the 30-Day Meal Plan, let's pretend that it's not just a schedule, but rather your guide to the land of health, where every day is a new adventure on your plate. Let's get on this culinary roller coaster!

Week 1: Discovering Taste

Days 1-7:
- Breakfast: Start with oatmeal topped with berries and seeds. Try a new combination each day - add banana and cinnamon, apple and almonds, pear and cardamom.

- Lunch: Chicken or tofu salad with lots of greens and vegetables. Experiment with dressings every day: olive oil with lemon, balsamic vinegar, and yogurt dressing.

- Dinner: Grill vegetables with a piece of salmon or chickpeas for a vegan option. Add different spices for variety, from Italian herbs to curry.

Week 2: Protein dip

Days 8-14:
- Breakfast: Protein pancakes with plain yogurt and fresh fruit. Change the fruit depending on the day.

- Lunch: Quinoa or buckwheat with vegetables and choice of protein-chicken, fish, beans. Play with combinations and sauces.

- Dinner: Light soups with seafood or legumes. Try a new soup recipe every day.

Week 3: Carbohydrate Exploration

Days 15-21:
- Breakfast: Smoothie with oatmeal, banana, nut butter, and cilantro or mint for freshness.
- Lunch: Whole grain pasta with a variety of sauces and vegetables. From classic pesto to tomato sauce with olives and capers.
- Dinner: Warm salads with quinoa, avocado, beets and nuts. Add a spoonful of goat cheese or tofu for protein.

Week 4: Vitamin Boost

Days 22-30:
- For breakfast: Scrambled eggs with avocado on whole wheat toast. Each day, add a new ingredient to the toast: tomatoes, arugula, and feta cheese.

- Lunch: Bowls with various ingredients: rice, vegetables, avocado, mango, shrimp, or tempeh. You can just experiment with combinations.

- Dinner: Baked chicken or squash with lots of greens. Use different herbs and spices each day to vary the flavor.

The key to a successful 30-day meal plan is flexibility and variety. Don't be afraid to change up your meals if you have a special craving or need certain ingredients for the day. Each meal must be satisfying, filling, and good for your body.

Recipes for breakfast, lunch, and dinner

Breakfast Recipes for 30 Days

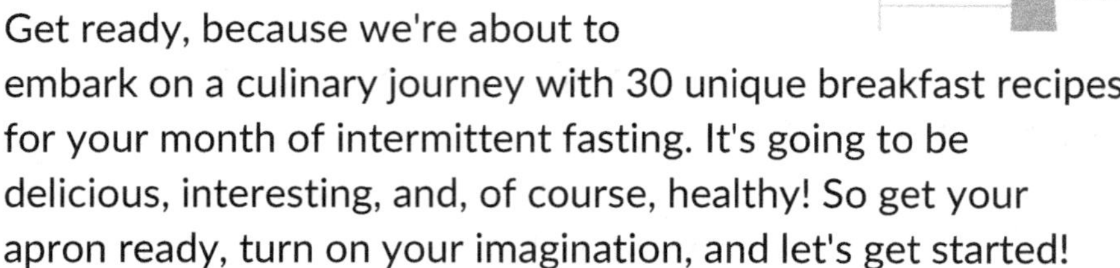

Get ready, because we're about to embark on a culinary journey with 30 unique breakfast recipes for your month of intermittent fasting. It's going to be delicious, interesting, and, of course, healthy! So get your apron ready, turn on your imagination, and let's get started!

Day 1: Smoothie Booster

- Blend a banana, a handful of spinach, a glass of almond milk, a spoonful of chia seeds, and some honey for sweetness. A green energy boost to boot!

Day 2: Avocado toast with eggs

- Toast whole wheat bread, mash half an avocado, top with a poached egg, and sprinkle with salt and pepper. A classic that never fails.

Day 3: Yogurt Fantasy

- Take Greek yogurt, add a spoonful of honey, a handful of nuts, and fresh berries. Simple but rich in flavor.

Day 4: Oatmeal with Apple and Cinnamon

- Boil oatmeal with water or milk, add a chopped apple, a pinch of cinnamon, and some nuts for crunch.

Day 5: Cottage cheese pudding with fruit

- Mix low-fat cottage cheese with egg, vanilla, and pieces of your favorite fruit. Bake until golden. Hello, childhood!

Day 6: Quinoa with Milk and Fruit

- Serve cooked quinoa with almond milk, fresh fruit, and a pinch of cinnamon.

Day 7: Protein Pancakes

- Mix protein powder with egg, banana, and milk until smooth. Fry pancakes and serve with berries.

Day 8: Shakshuka light

- Braised tomatoes with peppers and eggs are an oriental delight on your table. Serve with whole-grain bread.

Day 9: Hummus with Vegetables

- Spice up your morning with fresh vegetables and hummus. Quick, easy, and very healthy.

Day 10: Banana Oatmeal Muffins

- Bake ahead for a quick breakfast when it's a hectic morning.

Day 11: Turkey and Avocado Sandwich

- Whole grain bread, lettuce leaves, sliced turkey, and avocado. A protein and energy boost!

Day 12: Buddhist Bowl

- Chunks of fruit, nuts, and seeds with your choice of yogurt or honey topping.

Day 13: Scrambled eggs with veggies in a skillet.

It's like a rainbow on a plate: peppers, tomatoes, onions, spinach. Brown it all, then gently scramble a few eggs on top. Add a pinch of your favorite herbs and voila, your breakfast beauty is ready.

Day 14: Coconut Yogurt with Granola and Fresh Fruit Start your morning with some tropical flavor.

Coconut yogurt, granola for crunch, and a bunch of berries or mango chunks. It's not only delicious, it's energizing.

Day 15: Avocado and poached egg sandwich.

Toast whole wheat bread, mash avocado, and top with a poached egg. Sprinkle with flax or chia seeds for omega-3s.

Day 16: Green Smoothie Bowl.

A green smoothie made with spinach, kiwi, banana, and almonds will make your morning not only green but incredibly healthy.

Day 17: Feta and Olive Omelet.

Add a Mediterranean touch to your breakfast. Make a light and airy omelet with feta cheese and olives.

Day 18: Chia Pudding with Raspberries and Coconut.

Soak chia seeds in alternative milk overnight, then add raspberries and coconut flakes in the morning. It's like dessert for breakfast!

Day 19: Whole grain cheesecake with berry sauce.

Make it something sweet, but healthy. Make low-fat cottage cheese puffs with whole-wheat flour. Serve with a sugar-free berry sauce.

Day 20: Avocado toast with salmon and arugula.

A classic for those who like a saltier breakfast. Lean protein and healthy fats give you energy for the day.

Day 21: Quinoa porridge with apple and cinnamon.

Cook with water or vegetable milk, add apples and a little cinnamon for flavor.

Day 22: Smoothie with frozen blueberries, spinach, and Greek yogurt.

Let each sip be energized with freshness and goodness.

Day 23: Toast with ricotta and fresh figs.

Tender cheese and sweet figs on whole-grain toast are a feast on a plate.

Day 24: Oatmeal with pumpkin puree and pecans.

Start your morning with the flavors of fall, no matter the season.

Day 25: Shakshuka.

A little bit of the Middle East on your morning table. Tomatoes, peppers, onions, garlic, and eggs seasoned with zira and paprika. The perfect way to start the day with bright flavors and colors.

Day 26: Greek yogurt with cereal and honey.

Simple but incredibly delicious. Choose natural yogurt with no additives to get the most benefits.

Day 27: Turkey and avocado sandwich.

Use whole grain bread, add lettuce leaves, thinly sliced turkey, and sliced avocado for a breakfast that will keep you energized for a long time.

Day 28: Protein shake with raspberries, banana, and spinach.

Fill everything with non-dairy milk or water, add a scoop of protein powder for protein, and you've got the perfect breakfast on the go.

Day 29: Bulgur porridge with berries and nuts.

Bulgur is a great source of slow carbs. Add your favorite berries and a handful of nuts for extra nutrition and flavor.

Day 30: Avocado bowl with quinoa and egg.

Mix cooked quinoa and avocado slices in a bowl, then top with a poached or soft-boiled egg. Sprinkle with chia or flax seeds for an extra dose of omega-3s.

We hope these breakfast ideas inspire you to experiment and make your morning meal not only healthy but incredibly delicious. Remember, healthy eating is not boring and monotonous, but rather a variety of flavors that you can enjoy every day. Good luck in your culinary endeavors and let every morning start with something special!

Lunch Recipes for 30 Days

Just as the lunch bell rings at work, we move on to the most delicious part of the day - lunch! So get ready for 30 days of culinary discoveries that will make your lunches not only healthy but also incredibly appetizing as part of your intermittent fast.

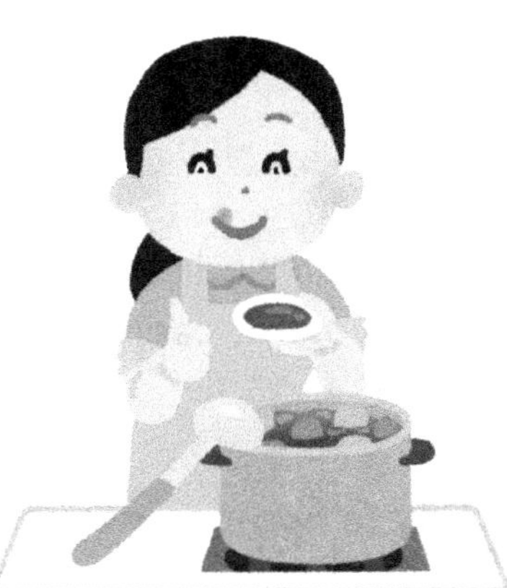

Day 1: Salad Nicoise

A classic with tuna, green beans, eggs, and olives. Dress with olive oil and lemon juice. It's like a mini vacation to the Côte d'Azur in your lunch hour.

Day 2: Lentil Soup with Coconut Milk

Warming and satisfying, the coconut milk adds an exotic

flavor. Serve with a slice of whole wheat bread for an extra treat.

Day 3: Chicken Breast with Quinoa and Avocado

Simple but flavorful. Roast the chicken breast with herbs, cook the quinoa in water, and slice the avocado. Drizzle with lemon juice and your lunch is ready.

Day 4: Vegetarian Poké Bowl

Rice or quinoa, marinated tofu, fresh cucumbers, carrots, avocado, and a slice of mango for sweetness. A dressing of soy sauce and sesame oil makes it perfect.

Day 5: Turkish Vegetable Fritters with Yogurt Sauce

Vegetable cutlets made from zucchini and carrots served with thick yogurt, garlic, and dill. It's like a little culinary tour of Istanbul.

Day 6: Shrimp Caesar

Substitute chicken for shrimp for a seafood version of your favorite salad. Don't forget the parmesan and whole-wheat croutons.

Day 7: Thai Salad with Mango and Shrimp

Toss together spicy shrimp, sweet mango, cucumber, and plenty of greens. Dress with lime and fish sauce for a real explosion of flavor.

Day 8: Sweet Potato Mashed Potato Soup

A warming and vitamin-packed soup with coconut milk and curry. Serve with crunchy whole wheat croutons.

Day 9: Stuffed Bell Peppers with Quinoa and Vegetables

Bake bell peppers stuffed with quinoa, black beans, corn, and tomatoes. Sprinkle with grated cheese or a vegan alternative.

Day 10: Couscous Salad with Vegetables and Feta Cheese

A light and refreshing salad to take to work. Toss couscous with cucumbers, cherry tomatoes, red onion, and diced feta cheese. Dress with olive oil and lemon juice for extra freshness.

Day 11: Japanese Miso Soup with Tofu and Seaweed

The perfect choice for those who want something light but hearty. Add miso paste, tofu, seaweed, and green onions, and you've got an umami-filled lunch.

Day 12: Vegetarian Black Bean Tacos

Bake corn tortillas and stuff them with black beans, avocado, red onions, and tomatoes. Add a pinch of cayenne pepper to spice things up.

Day 13: Mushroom and Spinach Risotto

An easy risotto over vegetable broth with the addition of mushrooms and spinach.

Sprinkle with parmesan or its vegan alternative before serving.

Day 14: Red Bean Salad with Corn and Avocado

Mix red beans, corn, diced avocado, red onion, and dress with lime and olive oil. Simple but very tasty.

Day 15: Bulgur with vegetable stew

Bulgur is a great alternative to traditional cereals, and combined with a vegetable stew of eggplant, peppers, and tomatoes, it makes a rich and healthy lunch.

Day 16: Boiled Beet and Goat Cheese Sandwich

Whole grain bread, boiled beets, goat cheese, and some greens. An easy and incredibly tasty way to satisfy your hunger.

Day 17: Light Chicken Salad with Pineapple

Toss chicken breast pieces with pineapple, cucumber, and pine nuts. Toss with a curried yogurt dressing for an exotic flavor.

Day 18: Grilled Buckwheat with Vegetables

Buckwheat is a great source of slow carbs. Add grilled vegetables like eggplant, bell peppers, and zucchini for a complete and healthy lunch.

Day 19: Spaghetti with Avocado Pesto

Make a pesto with avocado, basil, garlic, and olive oil for a light and healthy version of a favorite dish.

Day 20: Thai Chicken and Vegetables

Roast a chicken breast with mixed vegetables (carrots, broccoli, bell peppers) and add a sauce made with lime, soy sauce, and a little honey for sweetness.

I hope these ideas inspire you to try new combinations and not be afraid to experiment with lunch. After all, every lunch is an opportunity not only to be satisfied but also to get a little joy and pleasure out of eating. Remember that you can still enjoy variety and flavor while fasting; the main thing is to approach the choice of products and cooking with love and imagination.

Day 21: Courgette ribbons with pesto and shrimp

Light, airy, and incredibly tasty. The zucchini on the spiralizer replaces your pasta, and the shrimp adds protein. Top generously with homemade pesto.

Day 22: Quinoa, Avocado and Cherry Salad

This salad is a nutritional bomb. Add cherry tomatoes, diced avocado, and olives to the quinoa and dress with lemon juice and olive oil.

Day 23: Japanese Rolls with Vegetables and Quinoa

Forget white rice - quinoa also makes great rolls. Stuff them with fresh vegetables: avocado, cucumber, bell pepper, and add some wasabi for spice.

Day 24: Turkish Lentil Soup

Warming and very filling soup. Season with mint and paprika, and don't forget to add a scoop of yogurt when serving.

Day 25: Pumpkin and Chickpea Curry

A vegetarian version of an Indian classic. Serve with whole wheat rice or naan for a complete meal.

Day 26: Burrata Salad with Fresh Figs

The combination of mild burrata, sweet figs, aromatic basil, and balsamic cream is sure to please.

Day 27: Everyday Gazpacho Soup

The perfect choice for hot days. Refreshing, packed with vitamins, and easy to make.

Day 28: Ratatouille in Provence

A classic French dish rich in flavor and aroma. Serve with a slice of whole grain bread so you don't miss a drop of sauce.

Day 29: Warm Broccoli Salad with Garlic Sauce

Broccoli baked until golden and topped with a savory garlic sauce is both healthy and delicious.

Day 30: Carrot and Ginger Cream Soup

Carrots, ginger, coconut milk - and you have a dish with bright flavor and tons of benefits.

Dinner recipes for 30 days

The 30 days of lunch have flown by, and now it's time for dinner. Intermittent fasting dinners are your chance to end the day on a high note, with pleasure and health benefits. Let's make these evenings memorable with dinners you'll look forward to all day long!

Day 1: Light Arugula and Pear Salad

Start dinner with something fresh. Arugula, thinly sliced pears, blue cheese slices, and pecans are tossed in a honey mustard dressing.

Day 2: Grilled vegetables with tofu chunks

Marinate tofu in soy sauce with garlic and ginger,

then grill with eggplant, zucchini, and bell peppers. Simple, healthy, and delicious.

Day 3: Mashed Pea Soup with Mint

A light yet flavorful soup that is perfect for the evening. Add fresh mint for a refreshing accent.

Day 4: Steamed Teriyaki Chicken with Broccoli

Chicken marinated in teriyaki sauce served with steamed broccoli is a combination of flavor and goodness on one plate.

Day 5: Avocado, Mango and Shrimp Salad

An exotic combination of sweet mango, tender avocado, and spicy shrimp will make your dinner unforgettable.

Day 6: Pumpkin Cream Soup with Coconut Milk

Pumpkin soup with the addition of coconut milk and a hint of curry is a real warm hug after a long day.

Day 7: Courgette Spaghetti with Pesto and Tomatoes

An easy and healthy dinner that's also incredibly delicious. Replace traditional spaghetti with zucchini ribbons and add homemade pesto with cherry tomatoes.

Day 8: Baked Salmon with Asparagus

Simply wrap salmon and asparagus in foil and bake with lemon and herbs. It's quick, easy, and very elegant.

Day 9: Vegetarian Lasagna with Spinach and Ricotta

Who says dinner has to be boring? This lasagna is the perfect combination of flavor and goodness.

Day 10: Caesar Salad with Chicken Breast

The legendary salad can be made much healthier by opting for lean chicken and whole grain croutons.

Day 11: Turkey Schnitzel with Vegetable Stew

Tender steamed turkey cutlets served with a rich vegetable stew of eggplant, bell peppers, and tomatoes. Not only is this dish delicious, it's packed with all the vitamins and minerals you need.

Day 12: Quinoa Salad with Avocado and Black Beans

This is a great combination of textures and flavors. Quinoa provides complex carbohydrates, avocado adds healthy fats and black beans provide protein. Top with lime and olive oil for the perfect dinner.

Day 13: Quick Shakshuka.

A quick version of this classic dish. Tomatoes, peppers, onions, and eggs are cooked in a pan and served right away. A nice and easy way to end the day.

Day 14: Vegetable Curry with Lentils

A rich, nutritious, and flavorful dish that will leave you feeling full and warm. Serve with some brown rice or naan.

Day 15: Baked Yams with Quinoa and Greens

A yam baked until soft with a delicious topping of quinoa, green onions, cilantro, and a squeeze of lime. Simple, delicious, and very healthy.

Day 16: Warm salad with mushrooms and artichokes

Mushrooms and artichokes are pan-fried with garlic and herbs, then mixed with arugula or spinach. Dress it all with olive oil and balsamic vinegar.

Day 17: Red bean soup with smoked turkey

A hearty and flavorful soup that will warm you up on a cold evening. The smoked turkey will add a unique flavor.

Day 18: Fish in foil with vegetables

A favorite fish baked in foil with lemon, herbs, and any fresh vegetables. Simple, quick, and minimal dishes to wash.

Day 19: Teriyaki tofu with broccoli and carrots

A vegan dinner option full of flavor and benefits. Tofu is marinated in teriyaki sauce, fried until crispy, and served with steamed vegetables.

Day 20: Beet Salad with Goat Cheese and Walnuts

The rich flavors of beets and goat cheese complement each other perfectly, and walnuts add crunch. Tossed with olive oil and balsamic vinaigrette.

Day 21: Broccoli Cream Soup with Almonds

Try making broccoli cream soup by adding some grated almonds for creaminess and crunch. It's hearty, nutritious, and very comforting in the evening.

Day 22: Ratatouille with Quinoa

A classic ratatouille served with a side of quinoa will turn your dinner into a true French feast.

Day 23: Vegetarian Fajitas with Mushrooms and Bell Peppers
Sauté mushrooms, bell peppers, onions, and seasonings.

Wrap everything in whole-wheat tortillas for a delicious and easy dinner.

Day 24: Light Shrimp and Avocado Salad

Shrimp, avocado, fresh cucumber, and a squeeze of lime make the perfect summer salad. Dress with olive oil and enjoy every taste.

Day 25: Pasta and Vegetable Bolognese

Prepare pasta with a Bolognese sauce made from tomatoes, carrots, celery, and ling. It's rich in flavor and very comforting after a long day.

Day 26: Zucchini Boats Stuffed with Quinoa and Feta

Stuff zucchini with a mixture of quinoa, feta, tomatoes, and herbs, then bake in the oven. Simple but incredibly delicious.

Day 27: Warm Salad with Roasted Beets and Oranges

The combination of roasted beets with oranges and goat cheese is a real flavor treat. Serve with walnuts for added texture.

Day 28: Chicken Breast with Tomatoes and Olives

Bake a chicken breast with cherry tomatoes, olives, and capers. Add a little oregano for flavor. Simple but sophisticated.

Day 29: Vegetarian Bean and Corn Chili

Warm up with a hearty and flavorful vegetarian chili. Beans, corn, and lots of spices make this a memorable dinner.

Day 30: Couscous Salad with Vegetables and Pumpkin Seeds

Toss couscous with roasted vegetables and add pumpkin seeds for crunch. Dress with lemon juice and olive oil.

And so we come to the end of our 30-day culinary journey. I hope these dinner ideas inspire you to continue exploring the world of healthy eating.

And remember, every dinner is more than just a meal; it's a moment to savor and relax after a busy day. Experiment with ingredients and recipes, find your favorite dishes and make dinner your daily ritual of joy and self-care.

Helpful Tips

Here are a few more tips to make your 30-day cooking marathon not only rewarding but fun:

- Experiment with cuisines from around the world.

Immerse yourself in Italy one day with its famous pasta and pizza (yes, there are healthy options!), and the next day discover the flavors of Thailand with light soups and salads. The world's cuisines are an endless source of inspiration.

- Plan, but stay flexible.

Stock up on the right products ahead of time so you always have everything you need to prepare your planned meals. But if something suddenly doesn't go according to plan or you just want a change, no problem. The important thing is to stick to the principles of healthy eating.

- Emphasize fresh foods.

The fresher the food, the more nutrients it contains. Visit local markets, and choose seasonal fruits and vegetables - it is not only healthy but also add pleasure to the process of cooking and eating.

- Don't forget about hydration.

In addition to a balanced diet, it's important to drink plenty of clean water. It helps absorb nutrients, keeps your metabolism going, and helps you avoid overeating.

- Emphasize the pleasure of eating.

Healthy eating should not be associated with restriction and discouragement. Find joy in every meal and experiment with textures, flavors, and colors. This will make your 30-Day Eating Plan not only healthy but also incredibly satisfying.

- Use seasonal produce.

Not only are they tastier and healthier, but they will add variety to your diet throughout the year. Each season offers unique foods to experiment with in the kitchen.

- Play with spices and herbs.

Not only will they add flavor to your dishes, but they'll also provide additional health benefits. Turmeric, cinnamon, basil, mint - every spice will add flavor to your culinary masterpieces.

- Discover the benefits of multicookers and steamers.

These kitchen gadgets help you cook in the healthiest way possible, preserving all the nutrients in your food.

Make eating convenient:

- Preparation is your best friend.

By spending a few hours on the weekend prepping ingredients, you can quickly assemble complete meals during the week, saving time and nerves.

- Freezing is a lifesaver for busy days.

Many dishes and ingredients are perfect for freezing. You'll always have something healthy and delicious on hand, even when you don't have time to cook.

- Enjoy every moment:

- Invite friends and family. Sharing a meal not only strengthens relationships but also makes the meal more enjoyable and meaningful.

- Experiment with serving.

The visual appeal of a dish plays a big role in the enjoyment of a meal. A beautiful presentation can make even a simple dish special.

By following these principles, you can not only achieve your health and fitness goals but also enrich your culinary experience by discovering many new flavors and dishes. Let these 30 days be the beginning of your journey to a healthy and enjoyable lifestyle!

Chapter 7: A selection of meals that promote weight loss and improve metabolism.

Enjoy every meal! We've got plenty of ideas for meals that not only please your taste buds, but also help you lose weight and improve your metabolism.

Magic meals for slim and healthy

Easy Salads with Superfoods
Salads are more than just lettuce leaves. Add quinoa, avocado, nuts, chia seeds, and pomegranate seeds. Not only will these ingredients fill your body with nutrients, but their high fiber and healthy fats will help you burn fat.

Soups for heat and fat-burning

Vegetable soups made with low-fat broth or purees of broccoli, cauliflower, or squash are great choices for lunch or a light dinner. They'll keep you full, provide vitamins and minerals, and help you stay slim.

Protein Wonders

Protein is your staunchest ally in the fight for slimness. Chicken breast, turkey, or fish can be baked with herbs and vegetables for a protein-rich, low-calorie meal. This will help you build muscle mass and speed up your metabolism.

Smoothies for Energy and Metabolism

Smoothies based on greens with the addition of berries, bananas mangoes and coconut water or almond milk can be a great way to start the day. Add a scoop of protein powder or flaxseed to boost your metabolism and increase satiety.

Snacks that won't hurt your figure

Your best friends between meals are nuts, seeds, berries, and fruit. They'll help keep your energy and metabolism going and prevent you from overeating at main meals.

Cook smart

Use spices and herbs to add flavor without adding calories. Turmeric, ginger, chili, and cinnamon not only add flavor to your dishes but also speed up your metabolism and help you burn fat naturally.

So here's a series of recipes and tips to make every meal not only delicious but also good for your figure and health. Remember, the key to success is variety and moderation. Experiment with ingredients, combinations, and cooking methods to make your meals fun, healthy, and satisfying.

Don't forget that every meal is an opportunity to try something new and surprising, even with a healthy diet. Learning new recipes and techniques can become a hobby, turning each meal into an exploration of taste and benefits.

Keep exploring:

Let your imagination run wild with ingredients.

Don't be afraid to experiment with unusual combinations. Watermelon with feta and mint? Why not? Sweet potatoes with coconut milk and curry? Sounds like the perfect dinner. Experimenting will help you discover new flavors and make your diet more interesting.

Planning is the key to variety

Plan your menu for the week ahead, making sure to include a variety of foods and dishes. Not only will this help you maintain a healthy lifestyle, but it will also ensure that you're getting all the nutrients you need. Planning will also help you avoid making spontaneous decisions to snack on something that is not very healthy.

The social aspect of eating

Sharing a meal isn't just fun, it's also good for your mental health. Invite friends over for a healthy cookout. Not only will this strengthen relationships, but you can also share recipes and ideas for healthy eating.

Don't forget to enjoy

It's important to remember that food is not only a means of nourishment but also a source of pleasure. Remember to enjoy each meal and savor the taste and texture of foods.

Eating healthfully doesn't have to be boring or monotonous. Finding pleasure in eating well is the key to maintaining a healthy lifestyle over the long term.

Continuous learning 

The world of healthy eating is constantly evolving, and there is always something new to learn. Read books, watch documentaries, and subscribe to cooking blogs and healthy lifestyle channels. The knowledge and inspiration you gain will help you stay on track and add new ideas to your diet.

Remember that eating well is a journey of discovery and delicious adventure. Experiment, enjoy, and share your successes with your loved ones. You will not only reach your health and fitness goals, but you will also make your life brighter and more interesting.

Chapter 8: Vitamins and Foods to Boost Metabolism and Promote Weight Loss

Key vitamins and foods that promote weight loss.

A look at the world of vitamins and foods that not only make your diet healthier but also help you reach your weight loss goals. After all, proper nutrition isn't just about calories and exercise, it's also about micronutrients that play a key role in metabolic processes.

Vitamins and Foods to Help You Lose Weight:

So, are you ready to speed up your life? It's not about cars, it's about metabolism. If you want to get your inner motorist running like clockwork, get ready to take notes because I'm going to talk about vitamins that will get your metabolism into fifth gear.

Green light for speed

Vitamin D and Calcium

Not only for strong bones but also to support your metabolism. The combination of vitamin D and calcium helps your body burn fat more efficiently. Studies show that adequate vitamin D levels are associated with better weight loss. Sources: sunlight, fatty fish (salmon, sardines), eggs, and fortified foods.

Vitamin B12

This vitamin helps convert food into energy, which is essential for maintaining an active lifestyle and burning calories efficiently. It is found in meat, fish, dairy products, and fortified cereals.

Fiber-rich foods

Fiber helps you feel fuller for longer, which can help reduce your overall calorie intake. Oats, berries, vegetables, fruits, and whole grains are great choices.

Protein

Of course, we can't forget about protein. Not only does it help build muscle, which burns more calories even when you're resting, but it also speeds up your metabolism and keeps you feeling full longer. Include eggs, chicken breast, fish, cottage cheese, and beans in your daily diet to help you burn more calories.

Green tea and coffee

Green tea and coffee: Natural metabolism boosters. Caffeine gives you energy, while green tea is rich in antioxidants and contains catechins, which can help speed up metabolism and fat burning, especially in the belly area. So treat yourself to a cup of coffee or green tea without guilt.

Apple Cider Vinegar

While not a miracle cure, some studies show that apple cider vinegar may slightly accelerate weight loss by improving satiety and lowering blood sugar levels after a meal.
Iron

Your internal engine won't run at full speed without enough iron. This element helps carry oxygen to your muscles, keeping you energized and helping you burn fat. Load up on spinach, lentils, and red meat.

About Magnesium

Magnesium is like a little magic element, essential for hundreds of biochemical reactions in our bodies, including supporting the muscular and nervous systems, regulating blood sugar and blood pressure, and building bones and DNA. However, its absorption can depend on a variety of factors.

Vitamin B6 plays a key role in the absorption of magnesium.

 Studies have shown that vitamin B6 improves magnesium absorption by cells and may reduce magnesium excretion from the body. B6 is involved in many metabolic processes, and one of its functions is to help convert magnesium from its insoluble form to a soluble form that is more easily absorbed by the body

Other factors that affect magnesium absorption include

1. Phytates and fiber: Foods rich in phytates (such as certain grains and beans) can decrease magnesium absorption. It also appears that a high intake of dietary fiber may slightly interfere with magnesium absorption, although fiber is essential for digestive health.

2. Other Minerals: High doses of calcium, zinc, and iron taken at the same time as magnesium may compete for absorption, reducing the efficiency of absorption of each of these minerals.

3. Gut health: Because magnesium is absorbed in the intestines, digestive problems such as irritable bowel syndrome and inflammatory bowel disease can reduce the body's ability to absorb magnesium.

4. Alcohol: Regular alcohol consumption can decrease magnesium absorption and increase magnesium excretion.

To improve magnesium absorption, it is helpful to include foods rich in vitamin B6 in your diet. Together, magnesium and vitamin B6 not only improve each other's absorption but also help support a variety of functions in the body, including improving mood and reducing symptoms of premenstrual syndrome.

Magnesium and vitamin B6 make a great team when it comes to supporting nervous system health, reducing stress levels, and improving sleep.

Foods rich in magnesium:

- Green leafy vegetables (spinach, kale)
- Nuts (almonds, cashews)
- Seeds (pumpkin seeds, sunflower seeds)
- Legumes (black beans, lentils)
- Whole grains (buckwheat, quinoa)
- Avocados
- Bananas

Foods rich in vitamin B6

- Poultry (chicken, turkey)
- Fish (salmon, tuna)
- Potatoes and other root vegetables
- Fruits (except citrus), such as bananas
- Nuts and seeds

Recipes using a combination of magnesium and vitamin B6

<u>Avocado with tuna and sunflower seeds</u>

- Mash a ripe avocado with a fork, add canned tuna, a little lemon juice, and salt and pepper to taste.
- Sprinkle with sunflower seeds.
- This snack, rich in magnesium and vitamin B6, will help improve digestion and give you energy.

<u>Spinach Salad with Chicken and Almonds</u>

- Place fresh spinach leaves on the bottom of a plate.
- Arrange pan-seared chicken breast pieces on top and sprinkle with almonds.

- Dress with olive oil and lemon juice.
- This salad is not only delicious, but it also promotes better magnesium absorption thanks to the vitamin B6 in the chicken.

Quinoa with Black Beans and Avocado

- Cook quinoa according to package directions.
- Mix the cooked quinoa with the canned black beans, diced avocado, some chopped red onion, and herbs to taste.
- You can use olive oil with lemon juice as a dressing.
- This dish is a treasure trove of magnesium and vitamin B6.

Banana Smoothie with Almond Milk

- Blend a ripe banana, a glass of almond milk, a little honey or maple syrup for sweetness, and a pinch of cinnamon.
- The almond milk and banana provide magnesium and vitamin B6.

These simple and nutritious meals will help improve magnesium and vitamin B6 absorption, supporting your health and well-being.

Omega-3 fatty acids

These guys improve insulin sensitivity, reduce inflammation, and even help fight fat deposits.

Omega-3 fatty acids are essential fats that our bodies need to support heart health, brain health, and overall well-being.

They are not synthesized by the body, so they must come from food or supplements. Not only is it important to get enough omega-3s, but it's also important to promote better absorption. Here are some tips for improving omega-3 absorption:

What Improves Omega-3 Absorption:

1. Water soluble vitamins: Omega-3 is better absorbed in the presence of fats, especially fat-soluble vitamins such as vitamins D, A, and E. Eating foods rich in these vitamins or taking appropriate supplements can promote better omega-3 absorption.

2. Antioxidants: Omega-3 fatty acids can be oxidized if not protected by antioxidants. Therefore, including antioxidant-rich foods (berries, vegetables, fruits, nuts) in your diet can help preserve them and improve absorption.

3. Healthy fats: Combining omega-3s with other healthy fats, such as olive oil, avocados, and nuts, promotes better absorption.

What interferes with omega-3 absorption:

1. Trans Fats: The presence of trans fats in the diet can interfere with omega-3 absorption because they compete for the same enzymes in the metabolic pathway. Avoid foods with trans fats such as margarine, processed foods, and fried foods.

2. High omega-6 intake: Omega-6 and omega-3 compete for absorption in the body. Too much omega-6, which is common in the Western diet due to the high amount of vegetable oils, can interfere with omega-3 absorption. Aim for a balance between omega-6 and omega-3.

3. Alcohol and smoking: Excessive alcohol consumption and smoking can also negatively affect the absorption of omega-3 fatty acids.

Conclusion:

Improving omega-3 absorption depends largely on the overall composition of your diet and lifestyle. Remember, to maximize the benefits of omega-3s, it is important to eat a balanced diet rich in antioxidants, vitamins, and healthy fats, as well as a healthy lifestyle.

Including foods that contain fat-soluble vitamins and antioxidants in your diet will help improve the absorption of omega-3. It is also worth paying attention to the ratio of omega-6 to omega-3 intake, aiming to reduce the intake of the former and increase the latter. This will help avoid negative interactions between these fatty acids and promote better absorption of omega-3.

It is also important to remember that certain medications can interfere with the absorption of omega-3. If you are taking any medications, it is best to consult your doctor about their possible interaction with omega-3 supplements.

The following is an example of a balanced diet:

- Increase your intake of fatty fish such as salmon, sardines, and mackerel, which are excellent sources of omega-3 fatty acids.
- Add olive oil and avocados to salads and other dishes.
- Include nuts and seeds in your diet, especially flaxseed, which is rich in omega-3s.
- Eat more green leafy vegetables and antioxidant-rich fruits, such as berries and citrus fruits, to maintain good health and improve omega-3 absorption.

A healthy diet rich in omega-3s, supported by adequate vitamin and antioxidant intake, combined with avoiding unhealthy habits, will help maximize the positive effects of omega-3s on your health and well-being.

Vitamin C

Not only does it help fight colds, but it also activates the fat-burning process.

Vitamin C is a master of immune support and wound healing, and it also helps with iron absorption. If you want more of it in your diet, check out these foods - they're your vitamin bombs.
1- Rosehips are a true record-holder for vitamin C among natural sources.
2. Black currants - another superhero berry.
3. peppers - especially red peppers, which are not only delicious but also extremely useful.

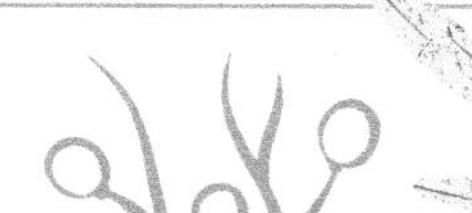

4. Kiwi - these small fruits contain a huge amount of vitamin C.
5. Green leafy vegetables - such as spinach, broccoli, and Brussels sprouts.
6. Citrus fruits - oranges, grapefruit, lemons and limes.
7. Papaya - a tropical fruit rich in vitamin C.
8. Strawberries - delicious and healthy, especially in season.
9. Guava - an exotic fruit, a leader in vitamin C content.
10. Mango - another tropical fruit packed with vitamin C.

Keep in mind that vitamin C is sensitive to heat processing, so many of these foods are best eaten raw to maximize their benefits.

Fill your body with these superfoods and you'll not only see the extra pounds disappear, but you'll also feel more energetic, happier, and healthier. Remember, eating right isn't a diet, it's a lifestyle. And like any good journey, it's important to savor every moment and every bite on your plate.

The benefits of chromium

Oh, talking about chromium is like opening Pandora's box in the world of nutrients, especially when it comes to interval fasting and the whole insulin resistance and unwanted weight gain thing. So grab your popcorn (but stop, we're fighting for our health here) and buckle up, let's get started!

What is chromium and why do we need it?

Chromium isn't just the shiny element that makes our cars look good. It's also a trace element that plays a key role in the metabolism of carbohydrates and fats. So if you want your metabolism to run like a Swiss watch, chromium is your best friend.

Interval fasting and chromium: Two stars in the health sky

When you practice interval fasting, your body begins to treat insulin, the hormone that regulates blood sugar levels, differently. And that's where chromium comes in! It's like it's telling our bodies, "Hey guys, let's make the most of this insulin!" This helps maintain normal blood sugar levels and reduces the urge to reach for sweets.

Fighting Insulin Resistance

Insulin resistance is when your body's cells start to ignore insulin's "call," which can lead to weight gain and, in the long run, more serious health problems. Enter chromium, and you've got a powerful helper that helps prevent all this trouble by keeping insulin sensitivity at the right level.

But how does it work?

When you eat, your blood sugar levels rise, and your body produces insulin to help use that sugar for energy. Chromium improves the action of insulin, which helps your body use sugar more efficiently and prevents it from being stored as unwanted fat.

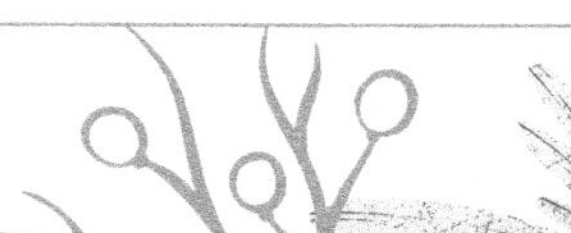

Where do I get it?

Chromium can be found in foods such as broccoli, whole grains, meat, and some fruits and vegetables. But honestly, to get the recommended dose, sometimes it's easier to use supplements, of course after consulting your doctor.

So, to summarize

Chromium is a kind of invisible hero in the fight for a healthy metabolism and weight control.

So, by adding these vitamins and foods to your diet, you are not only enriching your diet with all the essentials but also your blood sugar levels. When combined with intermittent fasting, it plays no small role in helping your body maximize the use of insulin and reduce cravings for snacks, especially sweets. It's like giving your metabolism a personal trainer and throwing in an appetite control assistant.

Among other things, adding chromium to your diet (after discussing it with your doctor, of course) can be an easy way to improve your body's response to insulin and thus reduce your risk of developing insulin resistance. This is especially important if you're doing intermittent fasting to not only lose weight but also to improve your overall health.

Interesting fact: Despite its invisibility in everyday life, chromium can have a noticeable impact on your well-being. From improved metabolism to more stable blood sugar levels, it is not just another supplement, but an important part of your health arsenal.

So if you've decided to try interval fasting, or if you're already on the path and looking for ways to optimize your results, don't forget to consider a supplement like chromium. It could be one of your best decisions on the road to a healthy lifestyle, a clear memory, and of course, controlling that funny number on the scale.

In the meantime, keep exploring, keep experimenting, and remember: self-care isn't selfishness, it's an investment in your future.

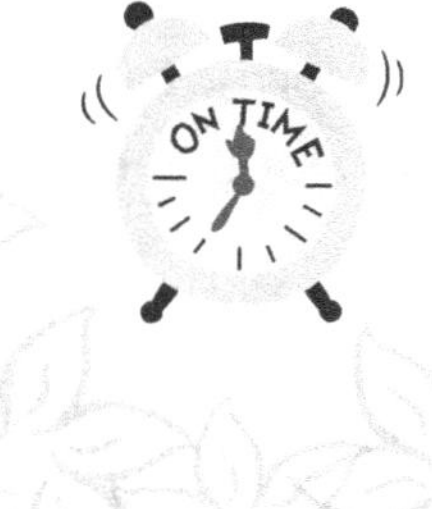

Chapter 9: Foods to Eliminate

A list of foods that cause insulin spikes and should be eliminated.

Now let's move on to the foods that can be a stumbling block on your path to a slimmer, healthier you. Proper nutrition is not only about what to eat but also what to avoid.

Foods to Avoid:

Sugar and Sweets

It's probably not news, but sugar is a major enemy not only of your figure but of your overall health. Sweet soda, candy, cookies, cakes, and other sweets cause blood sugar and insulin levels to spike, contributing to fat storage and insulin resistance.

White Bread and Flour Products

White flour products also contribute to blood sugar spikes. Choose whole grains, which have a lower glycemic index and more nutrients.

Fatty meats and sausages

Fatty meats and processed meats often contain saturated fats and trans fats, which can raise levels of "bad" cholesterol (LDL) and promote fat storage in the body.

Fast Food and Prepackaged Lunches

Fast food and convenience foods are high in calories, saturated fat, salt, and sugar, and low in nutrients. These foods not only contribute to weight gain but also to poor overall health.

Sugary drinks and alcohol

Sweet sodas, juice boxes, and alcoholic beverages are high in "empty" calories, which can easily exceed your daily energy intake and lead to weight gain.

Margarine and trans fats

Artificial trans fats found in margarine, certain types of cookies, crackers, and pastries can affect cardiovascular health and contribute to weight gain.

By avoiding these foods, you'll not only help control your weight, but you'll also improve your overall health, energy, and well-being. It's important to remember that healthy eating is not about rigid restrictions, but about making conscious choices to eat natural, nutritious foods that benefit your body.

Chapter 10: Metabolism and Memory Improvement

Tips for Accelerating Your Metabolism and Improving Cognitive Function

Let's dive into the topic of metabolic acceleration and cognitive enhancement. These two goals are interrelated, as brain health and metabolic efficiency directly affect each other. Here are some proven tips to help you stay physically and mentally energized.

Boost your metabolism:

1. Don't skip breakfast

Breakfast kick-starts your metabolism for the day. Choose foods rich in protein and fiber to keep you full and energized for longer.

2. Increase physical activity

Regular exercise, especially strength training, boosts your metabolism by increasing muscle mass, which burns more calories even when you're resting.

3. Drink plenty of water

Dehydration slows your metabolism, so it's important to drink plenty of water throughout the day. Cold water can speed up your metabolism even more because your body has to use energy to heat it.

4. Eat protein with every meal

Protein increases satiety and speeds metabolism through the thermic effect of food, the energy needed for digestion.

Improve Memory and Cognitive Function

1. Quality sleep

Nothing is more important to the brain than a good night's rest. Not getting enough sleep can seriously affect memory and learning ability.

2. Eat a healthy diet

Foods rich in omega-3 fatty acids (such as salmon), antioxidants (berries, nuts, green leafy vegetables), and B vitamins support brain health and help improve memory.

3- Mental exercises

Crosswords, puzzles, logic games, and learning new skills such as a foreign language or musical instrument help keep the brain sharp.

4. Regular breaks and relaxation

Stress takes a toll on the brain. Practicing meditation, deep breathing, or yoga can help reduce stress levels and improve cognitive function.

5. Social activity

Socializing with friends and family is not only fun but also good for the brain. Social interactions stimulate mental alertness and can help reduce the risk of dementia and depression. From maintaining social connections to participating in group activities or hobby clubs, it keeps your brain active, trains your memory, and promotes emotional well-being.

6. Exercise outdoors

Walking or exercising outdoors not only strengthens your body but also promotes better blood circulation, including to the brain. This improves cognitive function and helps combat stress.

7. Antioxidants in your diet

Foods rich in antioxidants, such as berries, dark chocolate, nuts, and green leafy vegetables, protect brain cells from free radical damage, keeping your brain healthy and improving your memory.

8. Omega-3 fatty acids

Omega-3 fatty acids, especially those found in fatty fish, flaxseeds, and walnuts, are important for brain health. They help improve memory, protect against cognitive decline, and may even improve mood.

9. Regular medical checkups

Certain diseases and conditions, such as diabetes, high blood pressure, and high cholesterol, can affect cognitive function. Regular medical monitoring and management of these conditions can help maintain mental clarity and memory.

By following these tips, you can not only speed up your metabolism and improve your physical health, but you can also significantly boost your cognitive abilities and improve your memory and concentration. Taking care of your body and brain is a comprehensive approach that will ensure not only your longevity but also your quality of life for years to come.

Understanding Metabolism and How Certain Foods Can Speed It Up

Hello Health Team! Today we're going to dive into the world of metabolism. Do you know that magical process that helps us turn pizza and salads into energy? It's like turning on your internal heater to automatically burn calories.
So let's figure out how to make that machine run faster and more efficiently.

What is thermogenesis?

Thermogenesis is the process by which our bodies produce heat. When we eat thermogenic foods, our bodies use more energy (read calories) to digest them. It's like throwing wood into a fireplace to start a fire.

Metabolism in 5 seconds

Think of your metabolism as a big factory that runs 24/7, processing everything you eat into energy that you use for everything from blinking to running marathons. And like any factory, its efficiency can fluctuate.

Premium fuel

Now that we know that our metabolism factory needs quality fuel, let's take a look at the foods that make it run like clockwork.

1. Protein:

Chicken, fish, tofu, legumes, and eggs are your new best friends. Proteins make your metabolism go into overdrive because your body needs more energy to digest them. This is called the thermic effect of food. The bonus is that you feel fuller for longer.

2. Spicy spices:

Do you like hot spices? Great!!! The capsaicin in peppers can give your metabolism a little boost. Add chili to your food and enjoy not only the flavor but also the little calorie-burning bonus.

3. Ginger and Cinnamon:

These spices not only add flavor to your food, but they can also increase thermogenesis a bit and control blood sugar levels.

4. Water:

Our metabolic factory can't run without water. Even mild dehydration can slow it down. Drink water, stay hydrated, and your metabolism will thank you.

5. Fruits and vegetables are our best friends:

Not only for the vitamins and minerals but also because the fiber in these foods makes your metabolism work harder to digest them. Broccoli, apples, pears - go for it.

6. Nuts and seeds-small but mighty:

The amino acids and healthy fats in nuts and seeds help speed up your metabolism. They're also great for filling you up, so you eat less and feel fuller longer.

How it works

When you eat thermogenic foods, it's like pushing your metabolism to work harder. Think of it like every time you eat a hot pepper or drink green tea, you're kicking your metabolic machine into overdrive. In the end, you're burning more calories, even when you're just sitting back and enjoying a cup of coffee.

It's important to remember:

There's no single magic product that will dramatically speed up your metabolism.

It's a combination of proper nutrition, exercise, and a healthy lifestyle. But adding these foods to your diet can help your "plant" work a little more efficiently.
So let's feed our metabolism quality fuel and enjoy the energy it gives us. And remember, taking care of your body is a marathon, not a race. Go for health and energy!

Bottom Line

Thermogenic foods are a cool way to speed up your metabolism and weight control. But as with anything, the key is variety and balance. You don't want to go overboard with spicy or caffeinated foods, but rather make these foods part of a balanced diet.

So if you want to get your metabolism going, you already know what to do. But remember, the best way to maintain your health and weight is a combination of proper diet, exercise, and healthy sleep. And thermogenic foods are just a small but nice bonus to your healthy lifestyle!

Chapter 11: Solutions to Stressful Overeating

Strategies for managing stress without resorting to overeating

Protect yourself from developing cognitive impairment as you age. So get-togethers with friends and family not only make your heart happy, they also make your brain happy.

By switching to solutions for stressful overeating, we enter a realm where emotions drive our eating more than physical hunger. Stressful overeating isn't about physiology, it's about psychology, and it's about finding ways to manage stress without turning to food as a means of self-soothing.

Here are some strategies to help you manage stress without overeating:

1. Identify triggers

Notice the times when you tend to turn to food for comfort. It could be a particular situation, emotion, or even time of day. Understanding your triggers is the first step to taking control of the situation.

2. Find alternative ways to relax

Instead of seeking solace in food, try other ways to relieve stress: take a walk in nature, meditate, do deep breathing, practice yoga, or enjoy a favorite hobby. These activities will help reduce stress without adding extra calories.

3. Exercise

Exercise not only helps you manage stress, it also improves your mood by releasing endorphins, the "happy hormones. Regular physical activity can be an effective strategy against stress-related overeating.

4. Keep a food and mood journal

By recording what and when you eat, as well as your emotions at the time, you can identify patterns of stress eating and work to change them.

5. Surround yourself with support

Sharing your concerns with friends, family, or a professional can help relieve stress. The support of loved ones is a powerful resource in the fight against stress and overeating.

6. Organize healthy meals

Make sure you always have healthy snacks on hand, such as vegetables, fruits, and nuts, so you don't resort to unhealthy snacking when you're stressed.

7. Practice mindful eating

Learn to eat slowly and mindfully, savoring each bite. This will help you feel full and avoid overeating.

By using these strategies, you can not only avoid stressful overeating but also improve your overall emotional well-being. Remember that stress is an integral part of life, but your attitude and how you deal with it make a big difference. By learning how to manage stress without turning to food for comfort, you'll take a big step toward a healthier lifestyle and improved well-being.

Keep exploring yourself

Everyone is unique, and what works for one person may not work for another. Don't be afraid to experiment with different strategies to find the ones that work best for you.

Set realistic goals

Don't strive for perfection or expect immediate results. Setting realistic goals and making lifestyle changes gradually is more likely to lead to long-term success.

Be kind to yourself

Treat yourself with compassion and understanding. If you snapped and turned to comfort food, don't punish yourself. Acknowledge the moment, learn a lesson, and move on.

Remember that each day gives you a new opportunity for choice and change. By managing stress without overeating, you will not only improve your physical health but also your emotional well-being and find more joy and fulfillment in life.

Chapter 12: Ideal Foods for Breakfast, Lunch, and Dinner

Examples of Balanced Meals for Each Meal of the Fasting Diet

Now let's move on to something more delicious and satisfying: the perfect foods and meals for breakfast, lunch, and dinner that will help you stay within the limits of interval fasting while still enjoying each meal.

Breakfasts that give you energy

Start the day with a meal rich in protein and fiber to jumpstart your metabolism and keep you feeling full for longer.

- Try oatmeal over water or milk with berries and nuts. Oatmeal is a great source of complex carbohydrates and fiber, while berries and nuts add vitamins and healthy fats.

- Omelet with vegetables. Protein and fiber are your best morning friends. Add spinach, tomatoes, and any other veggies you like to your omelet.

Lunches that keep your rhythm going

In the middle of the day, you need to keep your energy up without overloading your stomach. The ideal lunch is balanced and not too heavy.

- Salad with chicken or fish. Protein and fresh vegetables = the perfect lunch combination. This dish will provide you with energy and nutrients without causing drowsiness.

- Quinoa or buckwheat with vegetables. Complex carbohydrates and fiber give you the energy you need for the second half of the day.

Dinner for recovery

In the evening, it is important to prepare the body for recovery, so dinner should be light but nutritious.

- Try steamed salmon with steamed broccoli. The omega-3 fatty acids in the salmon support your heart and brain, and the broccoli provides fiber.

- Warm quinoa salad with avocado and fresh vegetables. Light and nutrition is what you want for dinner.

A word about appetizers

If your intermittent fasting schedule allows room for snacks, choose foods that will keep your energy levels up without causing blood sugar spikes.

- Nuts and seeds. A small handful of nuts can satisfy your hunger. Fresh veggies with hummus. A classic healthy snack. Remember, eating right isn't just about choosing healthy foods, it's also about savoring your food and enjoying every meal.

Chapter 13: Contraindications to Intermittent Fasting

While IG is a cool thing, it's not for everyone. Here's who should avoid it:

1. People who are emaciated:
If you're already underweight or have a very low body fat percentage, fasting isn't good for you. Your body will start eating its proteins, which is not cool at all.

2. If you're too young:
For those under 18, fasting can seriously affect development and growth. Toddlers and teenagers need adequate nutrition for normal growth and development, especially during puberty.

3. Pregnant and lactating mothers:
Expecting a baby or breastfeeding? Starvation is not your choice. A developing baby needs all the nutrients for healthy growth.

4. People with anorexia nervosa:
If you are anorexic or prone to anorexia, fasting may make the problem worse. Anorexia is a serious mental disorder, and restricting food will only make it worse.

5. People with certain medical conditions:
If you have gout or other specific nutritional or metabolic conditions, it's best to consult your doctor before starting a fast.

Most importantly, fasting should not become an excuse to overeat on other days or a way to punish yourself for food "sins. It is a tool that can help in some cases, but it is not for everyone and not always. When in doubt, it's best to consult a doctor.

Interval fasting is not just a diet, it's a lifestyle. But like any lifestyle, it should be approached intelligently and with respect for your body. Remember, the key to successful IG is flexibility, listening to your body, and common sense. Start gently, finish wisely, and may your journey be a happy and healthy one!

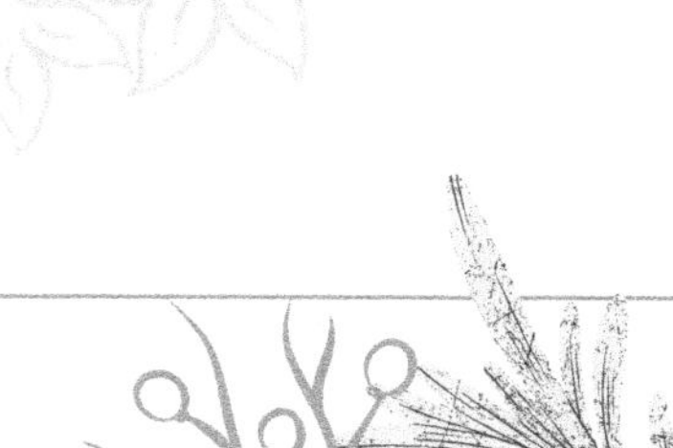

Conclusion

To summarize and encourage readers to get on the road to a healthy lifestyle through interval fasting.

Well, here we are, we have reached the finish line of our journey through the world of interval fasting and healthy living. Let me summarize a few things and give you a few pointers before you embark on your adventure.

 So what have we learned?

- Interval fasting is not just a diet, it's a lifestyle. Not only will it help you lose excess weight, but it can also improve your overall health, speed up your metabolism, and even increase your energy levels.

- The key to success is proper nutrition. Nutritious foods, balanced meals, and eating in moderation will help you get the results you want and feel better about yourself.

- Physical activity and quality sleep are your true allies in achieving a healthy lifestyle.

- Stress management and finding alternative ways to relax are important to avoid emotional overeating and maintain your mental balance.

A word of advice for the journey

Remember that any lifestyle change is a marathon, not a sprint. Don't look for immediate results; be patient and consistent. Interval fasting can be your true guide to health, but only if you follow its principles wisely and according to your individual needs.

- Listen to your body. It will tell you when it's time to eat and when it's time to rest.

- Experiment. Do not be afraid to try new foods and recipes. Variety is the key to a healthy, interesting diet.

- Enjoy every moment. A healthy lifestyle isn't just about restrictions-it's about enjoying what you're doing for your body and soul.

And remember, the journey to a healthy lifestyle is one of discovery and adventure. Along the way, you'll learn a lot about yourself, how your body works, and what's important for your well-being.

So, on to new horizons and accomplishments! Interval fasting and healthy living await you. Good luck on this exciting journey, and remember that you are not alone you will always have support, advice, and inspiration to help you reach your goals.

Apps

Frequently Asked Questions (FAQs) about IF for Women Over 50

Ida addresses the questions that hang in the air like fluffy clouds over the heads of women over 50 when they hear about Interval Fasting (IF). It's so important to have clear answers, especially when it comes to health and wellness.

1. "Can IF be beneficial at my age?"

Absolutely, yes! IF can be a great way to maintain a healthy weight, improve metabolism, and even boost energy levels. But, as with any age, it's important to approach this method wisely, taking into account individual needs and health.

2. "Won't IF affect my bone mass?"

This is an important question because the risk of osteoporosis increases with age. So far, there are not many studies showing a direct link between IF and bone loss. However, it is important to make sure you get enough calcium and vitamin D in your diet. And, of course, don't forget about exercise, including strength training.

3. "What about energy? Won't I feel tired?"

Many women find that, on the contrary, they feel a burst of energy after adjusting to IF. But!

The first few weeks can be challenging as your body adjusts. Drink plenty of water, remember to eat balanced meals, and listen to your body. If you feel tired, it may be worth adjusting your IF regimen.

4. "Can I combine IF with my regular exercise?"

Absolutely! Many people find that exercising on an empty stomach in the morning helps them feel more energetic. The key is to monitor how you feel. If you feel weak or dizzy during your workout, it may be worth adjusting your workout time or eating window.

5. "Do I need to take breaks from doing IF?"

Some experts recommend taking breaks from interval fasting from time to time to give your body a rest. This may be especially true for women over 50, given possible hormonal changes and body needs. Listen to your body and consult your doctor if necessary.

Hopefully, these answers will help dispel some doubts and encourage you to explore interval fasting further. Remember, every woman is unique and the key to success is personalization.

Resources for Further Reading and Support (Books, Websites, Forums) + health tracker

Oh, if you're ready to dive deeper into the world of interval fasting or any other aspect of healthy living, I have a treasure trove of information for you! So arm yourself with bookmarks, tablets, or old-fashioned notepads, and start taking notes!

Deep Dive Books:

1. "Eat Stop Eat by Brad Pilon - a classic of the IF genre that gives great insight into the basics and benefits of the practice.

2. "The Complete Guide to Fasting by Dr. Jason Fung - an in-depth study of interval fasting from a scientific perspective, plus practical advice.

3. "The Obesity Code, also by Dr. Fung - here the author uncovers the roots of obesity and offers solutions through proper nutrition and IF.

Websites for your daily dose of inspiration:

1. DietDoctor.com - tons of articles, research, and personal stories about IF and low-carb diets.

2. AuthorityNutrition.com - science-based articles on nutrition, including interval fasting, with reviews of the latest research.

3. Reddit - r/intermittentfasting - a community of like-minded people where you can find motivation, share experiences, and get answers to your questions.

Forums and social media for support and motivation:

1. MyFitnessPal - a great app for tracking food and exercise where you can also find a community of support.

2. Facebook Groups - there are tons of interval fasting groups where members share their successes, recipes, and tips.

3. Instagram and YouTube - many bloggers and wellness experts regularly post helpful content, including success stories, motivational videos, and even live discussions.

Remember, the wellness journey is a marathon, not a sprint. The more you learn, the easier it will be to find the approach that best fits your unique needs and goals. Explore, experiment, and don't be afraid to ask for community support. We're all in this together, so let's support each other on this amazing journey to better health and happiness!

How do I get a health tracker?

To keep track of how you eat, how much water you consume, and your physical activity, a health tracker has been created for you. To download and print the file, email me at
juliyajones1@gmail.com
Please include your name, book title, and the keyword "Health Tracker" and I will send you the download link.

About the Author

Julia Jones: The Journey to Health and Longevity through Interval Fasting

In a world where every day brings something new in the field of diet and nutrition, Julia Jones' story stands out for its depth and inspirational power. Her book, Interval Fasting for Women After 50, not only offers a fresh perspective on nutrition and self-care but also demonstrates how a scientific approach can lead to real changes in health and well-being.

From personal experience to a scientific approach

Julia Jones crossed the threshold at age 50 and faced common challenges: weight gain, declining overall health, and decreased energy. Dissatisfied with standard recommendations and searching for more effective solutions, she immersed herself in the world of scientific research and medical evidence. Thus began her journey into intermittent fasting, a method validated by science as a way to not only lose weight but also improve overall health.

Benefits for Mind and Body

 Julia Jones found that intermittent fasting had many positive effects on the body. In particular, she noticed improvements in heart function and memory clarity, which is especially important for women her age. The most significant discovery, however, was that through intermittent fasting, Julia was able to overcome insulin resistance, a problem that had long eluded her.

Scientific basis and personal experience

In her book, Jones shares not only her personal experience but also a comprehensive analysis of the scientific research that supports the effectiveness of intermittent fasting. She convincingly demonstrates how this method not only promotes weight loss, but also improves metabolism, reduces the risk of cardiovascular disease, and improves cognitive function.

Inspiration for women

 Julia Jones' book has been an inspiration to thousands of women looking for ways to improve their health after 50. She not only offers an effective plan of action but also emphasizes the importance of an individualized approach that recognizes the uniqueness of each body.

More than diet

 Julia Jones has proven that intermittent fasting is not just a diet, but a lifestyle that promotes deep self-discovery and understanding of one's body. Her method emphasizes the importance of listening to oneself and adapting conventional recommendations to individual needs and circumstances. Jones encourages women to pay attention not only to their diet, but also to their emotional well-being, stress levels, and sleep quality, emphasizing their role in achieving overall health and happiness.

Support and Community

Through her publications and speaking engagements,

Julia has created a strong support network for women facing similar challenges. Her book not only informs, but also brings women together, providing a platform to share their experiences, successes, and challenges on their journey to a healthy lifestyle after 50.

Practical and accessible approach

An important feature of Jones' work is her commitment to making intermittent fasting understandable and accessible to everyone. She breaks down complex medical concepts into simple and practical advice, making healthy living an achievable goal for every woman.

Bottom Line

 Julia Jones, through her book Interval Fasting for Women After 50, demonstrates that taking care of one's health is a comprehensive approach that requires attention to nutrition, physical activity, mental well-being, and emotional well-being. Her work is not just a nutrition textbook, but a life-changing guide that shows how proper nutrition, scientifically proven methods, and personal experience can work together for health and longevity. Julia Jones has become a true inspiration to women around the world who sincerely want to change their lives for the better.

Enjoyed the journey with "Intermittent Fasting for Women Over 50"?
I'd love to hear your thoughts! Please consider leaving a review to share your experience and help others discover the benefits.
Thank you for your support! Warm regards, Juliya Jones